MW01094200

Schuessler's

TISSUE SALTS REDISCOVERED

THE 21ST CENTURY GUIDE TO SELF-HEALING

By Lisa Strbac
LCHE BSc(Hons)

Schuessler's
TISSUE SALTS REDISCOVERED
THE 21ST CENTURY GUIDE TO SELF-HEALING

www.lisastrbac.com

For everyone who seeks the truth

Contents

"The twelve mineral salts are, in a very real sense, the material basis of the organs and tissues of the body and are absolutely essential to their integrity of structure and functional activity. Experiments prove that the various tissue cells will rapidly disintegrate in the absence of the proper proportion of these salts in the circulating fluid. Whereas the maintenance of this proportion insures healthy growth and perpetual renewal.

These mineral salts are, therefore, the physical basis of all healing. Regardless of the school employed, if these are absent from the blood and tissues, no permanent cure is possible."

Dr. Chas W. Littlefield

An introduction to this book

Hello,

My first experience of tissue salts was a little bit magical. Having recently learnt about them at homeopathy college, my husband had returned from a dentist appointment saying he had a cavity and was to go back for a filling in a few weeks. It was serendipitous timing that I'd heard that the tissue salts Calc Fluor and Calc Phos could help remineralise teeth, so I told him to take them for a month or two and delay his follow up. When he did go back to have his filling, the dentist declared they could no longer find the cavity. This is the power of these little tissue salts.

Fast forward to now and I've been repeatedly asked, in my work as a homeopath, to write a book on tissue salts for the home user. Tissue salts are an amazing place to begin in one's holistic health journey because they're simple, inexpensive and effective. While this book is intended to be a standalone guide for anyone new to natural remedies, I have also made some brief references to how they differ from homeopathic remedies (as this is a question I have been asked many times when delivering my homeopathy courses). Tissue salts are great for any beginner because they are prescribed based on physical symptoms rather than the wider 'like cures like' homeopathic principle. With 12 core tissue salts, compared to the thousands of homeopathic remedies, it is by far a simpler and less overwhelming place to begin.

There's lots of texts on the history of tissue salts, in particular as to whether they are 'homeopathic' remedies. Schuessler, the founder of tissue salts, initially titled his original work 'An Abridged System of Homeopathic Therapeutics.' However, as noted by Roger Savage in the foreword to 'Schuessler's Twelve Tissue Remedies' by Boericke & Dewey, by the end of Schuessler's life and career he had denied any connection with homeopathic principles, instead claiming that tissue salts are '**not based on homeopathic law but upon physiological chemical processes that take place within the organism.'**

My personal view is that, whatever label may be attributed to them, they are much needed right now. I believe that the state of our world is far more toxic than it was hundreds of years ago when Hahnemann, the founder of homeopathy, and Schuessler were alive and we now need many more tools at our disposal. And more importantly there can be significant health benefits from using tissue salts.

Whilst there are many (great) books on tissue salts most are the original old texts. I wanted to create something a little bit different... a small but simple guidebook that brings each one to life with visual graphics. I hope you enjoy.

Lisa Strbac

Homeopath LCHE BSc(Hons) & Integrative Health Coach

Schuessler's
Biochemical Tissue Salts

Doctor Willhelm Heinrich Schuessler (1821-1898) was a prominent German physician and biochemist known for his pioneering work in the field of biochemistry and his development of the concept of tissue salts, also known as cell salts, mineral salts or Schuessler salts.

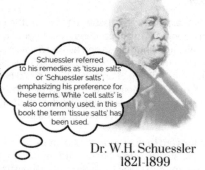

Schuessler referred to his remedies as 'tissue salts' or 'Schuessler salts', emphasizing his preference for these terms. While 'cell salts' is also commonly used, in this book the term 'tissue salts' has been used.

Dr. W.H. Schuessler
1821-1899

The fundamental principles of Schuessler's tissue salt theory are that:

- When the human body is reduced to ashes there remain only 12 tissue salts.
- It is these 12 tissue salts that are crucial for the body's survival.
- Any disease indicates an imbalance of these tissue salts within the body's cells.
- Health can be restored by supplying the required tissue salts to the body.

Schuessler believed that highly diluted preparations of specific tissue salts could be used to stimulate the body's self-healing mechanisms and restore balance within the cells. Schuessler provided humanity with a simple and non-toxic way to address imbalances and support the body's natural healing processes.

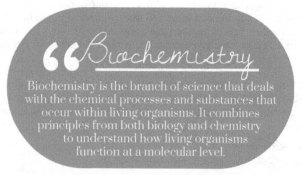

" Biochemistry

Biochemistry is the branch of science that deals with the chemical processes and substances that occur within living organisms. It combines principles from both biology and chemistry to understand how living organisms function at a molecular level.

The Tissue Salt Theory

 Health and disease are determined by the presence or absence of certain tissue salts within the body's cells.
Schuessler believed that when these tissue salts are deficient or imbalanced, it can lead to various health problems. By identifying and replenishing these deficient tissue salts, one could restore balance and promote healing.

 Each tissue salt has a specific function or role within the body's cells.
For example, Calc Fluor is essential for maintaining the elasticity of connective tissues, while Kali Phos is involved in cellular energy production. By understanding the functions of each tissue salt, one could determine which salts are needed to address specific health concerns.

 Tissue salts must be present in the correct proportions and distributed evenly throughout the body's cells in order to maintain health.
Imbalances or deficiencies in the distribution of these salts can disrupt cellular function and lead to disease. By ensuring the proper distribution of tissue salts, one could support overall health and well-being.

 Schuessler advocated for the use of highly diluted forms of tissue salts.
These would help to stimulate the body's natural healing processes. He believed that these highly diluted preparations could be more effective than larger doses of the same salts, as they work on a subtle energetic level to restore balance within the body's cells.

 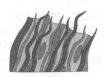

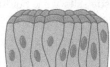

How are Tissue Salts made

Tissue salts are prepared using a specific method that involves grinding and diluting mineral compounds. Here's an overview of the process:

1. Selection of Mineral Compounds: Schuessler identified 12 mineral compounds that he believed to be essential for cellular health.
2. The crude mineral compounds are individually triturated, or ground, along with lactose, in a mortar and pestle. The ratio is one part of the mineral to 9 parts of lactose.
3. One part of the triturated mineral compound is then added to 9 parts of lactose and again triturated to give a 2x potency.
4. This process can be repeated indefinitely but, in practice, 6x potency is most frequently used. This means it has gone through the dilution process 6 times. This dilution process is essential for enhancing the therapeutic potency of the tissue salts. It is believed that this potentisation process activates the energetic properties of the mineral compounds, making them more effective in supporting cellular health.
5. Formulation: The potentised mixture is typically formed into small tablets, granules or sprays which are designed to be taken orally. Tissue salts are absorbed directly into the bloodstream via the mouth, rather than being assimilated via the digestive system.

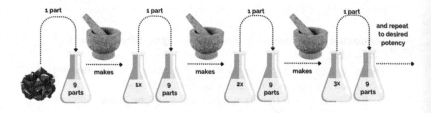

Even though tissue salts are highly diluted, they do still contain a minute material dose of the original minerals because they do not exceed Avogadro's number (this is a law of chemistry which states there is a limit to any dilution that can be made without losing the original substance altogether. This limit corresponds to homeopathic potencies of 12C).

There are various opinions on how tissue salts 'work' but they are generally believed to exert a therapeutic influence on the body's cells, aligning with Schuessler's principles of biochemistry.

How to choose & dose

Tissue salts are an amazing place to start with home prescribing. They are chosen based on the PERCEIVED DEFICIENCIES and PHYSICAL symptoms of the individual.

HOW TO CHOOSE A TISSUE SALT:

1. Identify Symptoms: Note physical symptoms like fatigue, digestive issues or skin problems.
2. Find your health issue in the symptoms index on pages 35-39 of this book - if it is not listed choose the most similar issue.
3. Look up each Tissue Salt listed to the description in this book. Understand each salt's functions; for instance, Calc Fluor aids elasticity, while Kali Phos helps with anxiety.
4. Match Symptoms: Compare your symptoms to each salt's indications, selecting the one that aligns best. If you feel that more than one Tissue Salt is a good match then it is fine to take more than one.
5. Consider Combinations: Sometimes, a blend of tissue salts is more effective.
6. Consult a Practitioner: If uncertain or dealing with complex issues, seek guidance from a qualified practitioner knowledgeable about tissue salts. They can offer tailored advice based on your needs.

DOSING GUIDELINES:

- CHRONIC OR LONG TERM ILLNESS: Take tissue salts frequently throughout the day. This can range from 2 to 6 times daily, depending on the severity of symptoms. If unsure, start with twice a day. Use for at least 1 to 3 months for optimum results.
- ACUTE ILLNESS: For sudden or acute illnesses, take up to every 15 minutes throughout the day. When the acute episode is over, usually after 24-72 hours, stop taking.
- NUMBER OF PILLS: It can vary depending on the specific manufacturer but generally take 1-4 tablets.
  Children should take half dose and infants a quarter dose.

POTENCY:

- Tissue salts are prescribed in a low potency, usually 6x (though other potencies like 3, 9 or 12x may also be used)

 Please be sensible and use your judgement. If healing is not happening or it is a medical emergency, please seek help from an appropriate healthcare professional.

FAQs

How do tissue salts differ from mineral supplements?
While standard mineral supplements give the body a material dose of the minerals, Schuessler believed that the micro-doses of tissue salts were more readily absorbed into the bloodstream and the body's tissues and cells than the larger material doses found in mineral supplements.

How do tissue salts differ from homeopathy in how they are made?
Even though tissue salts are highly diluted, they do still contain a minute material dose of the original minerals, whereas homeopathic remedies (once higher than a 12c) only contain the energetic imprint of the original substance.

How do tissue salts differ from homeopathy in terms of selection?
In selecting tissue salts, we focus on matching specific mineral deficiencies or imbalances within the body's cells to the symptoms and health concerns we wish to address. Each tissue salt has distinct properties and functions, making it easier to choose based on the specific symptoms present. On the other hand, homeopathic remedies are selected based on a broader principle of 'like cures like,' where a substance that causes symptoms in a healthy person is used to treat similar symptoms in a sick person. This means that homeopathic remedies may be chosen based on a broader set of symptoms and characteristics, rather than targeting specific mineral imbalances as with tissue salts.

Can I self prescribe tissue salts for chronic or long term health issues?
Yes, tissue salts can be self prescribed for long term health issues. For optimum results, take for at least 1-3 months.

I heard there are more than 12 tissue salts?
Though not widely known, there are additional salts (some say an additional 15 and others 21) which were later discovered by the followers of Schuessler. These additional salts are applied like the basic tissue salts but for more specific uses.

Can I take tissue salts if I am taking conventional medication, supplements or homeopathy?
Yes.

FAQs

Will tissue salts help with all conditions?
Tissue salts can help with MANY conditions. However, if the root cause of the health issue is due to an emotional disturbance then the health issue may return once the tissue salts have been stopped. For example, consider the case of someone who has 'never been well since' a sudden shock and has entered an exhausted and anxious state. While Kali Phos might be the tissue salt that helps them most on a day to day level, it is not necessarily getting to the root cause. Whereas a homeopathic remedy that can act on a deeper emotional level in a high potency might be able to clear the energetic disturbance so that the health issue does not return.

Can I take all 12 tissue salts at once?
While a combination of 12 can be helpful, it is recommended to select the specific tissue salts based on the individual's current presenting symptoms for a more targeted effect.

Can I take more than one tissue salt at a time?
Yes more than one tissue salt can be taken at the same time. In general 2-5 tissue salts can be taken at the same time for long-standing issues. It is also possible to buy pre-made combinations (as shown in pages 42-47).

Are tissues salts safe in pregnancy, while breastfeeding and for infants?
Yes, tissue salts are safe, non-toxic, have no side effects and are safe for all the above. Give children half the adult dose and infants a quarter.

Can I make my health worse by taking tissue salts?
No. It is almost impossible to make a health condition worse by taking tissue salts.

Can I get tissue salts in a non-lactose formulation?
Whilst traditionally made with lactose, there are lactose-free preparations available.

Where can I buy tissue salts from?
Tissue salts are available across the world, check www.lisastrbac.com for details of stockists.

The Twelve Tissue Salts

The Twelve Tissue Salts

Summary

Tissues salts are generally numbered though the order can vary by region. This book has used alphabetical sequence.

Tissue Salt	Description
Calc Fluor	Restores elasticity, strengthens teeth and bones
Calc Phos	Provides nutrition, builds cells, bone health, supports bone growth, rehabilitates
Calc Sulph	Cleanses blood, dissolves discharges, eliminates infections, heals wounds
Ferrum Phos	First Aid remedy, use in first stage of illness, anti-inflammatory, oxygen transporter
Kali Mur	Decongestant, detoxifier, supports glands, cleanses lymph
Kali Phos	Nerve and brain nutrient, calms nerves, anxiety, fatigue
Kali Sulph	Conditions skin and mucus membranes, late stage infections, oxygen carrier
Mag Phos	Cramps, pain, relaxes nerves and muscles
Nat Mur	Balances fluid, use for any watery discharges, dryness, dehydration
Nat Phos	Acid neutraliser and balancer
Nat Sulph	Detoxifies, eliminates fluid, cleanses liver
Silica	Skin and tissue cleanser and conditioner, helps with hair loss

Calc Fluor
Number 1 for elasticity

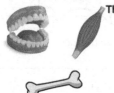

This salt is concentrated in:
Surface of bones
Enamel of teeth
Elastic fibres and skin
Muscle tissues
Connective tissues
Walls of blood vessels

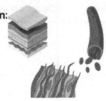

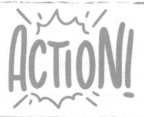

Elasticity
Flexibility
Strength

GENERAL ACTION & KEYNOTES

- A disturbance in the equilibrium of this salt can cause relaxation of elastic fibres and connective tissues creating issues such as enlarged veins, piles and sluggish circulation
- Strengthens surface of bones and joints
- Helps with weak teeth and decay
- Helps with weak ligaments including hypermobility and excessive bendiness
- Useful for hard nodules
- Heals prolapses, varicose veins, piles, fissures
- Helps with cracked skin

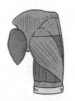

relaxed or hard elastic fibres

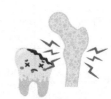

strengthens bones & teeth

weak ligaments

prolapses

humidity

massage

Person's symptoms are hindered by:
Humidity
Damp

Person's symptoms are helped by:
Massage
Warmth

Calc Fluor

Restores elasticity, strengthens bones & teeth enamel

Body Part / System		Symptoms
Mind		depression indecision
Head		lumps swellings sinusitis
Eyes		cataracts
Ears		n/a
Mouth		teething tooth decay inflamed gums coldsores burning or tickling in throat
Digestive system		constipation itching of rectum piles (hemorrhoids)
Respiratory system		croup tickling in larynx
Kidneys/bladder		uterine prolapses
Skin, blood & hair		skin - restores elasticity cracked skin & heels wrinkles stretchmarks hard swellings or nodules hair loss varicose veins
Bones, joints & ligaments		strengthens bones & weak ligaments inflammation of knee joints cracking in joints injured ligaments or sore muscles hypermobility arthritis
Female		heavy menses post partum haemorrhages

Calc Phos
Number 1 for bone health

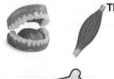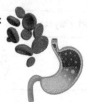

This salt is concentrated in:
Bones
Teeth
Connective tissues
Blood cells
Digestive juices

ACTION!

Provides nutrition
Builds cells
Bone growth
Rehabilitates

GENERAL ACTION & KEYNOTES:
- Essential for growth and nutrition, promotes healthy cellular activity
- Stimulates cell production
- Increases vitality - acts like a general restorative tonic for use after acute illnesses
- Restores weak organs and tissues
- Bone health
- Healthy teeth formation
- Important during periods of rapid growth such as in childhood and during puberty
- Increases vitality in the elderly
- Nutrient for blood

builds cells

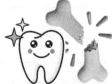

strengthens bones & teeth

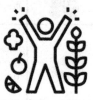

growth & nutrition

restorative tonic

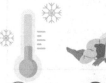

 cold

 rest

Person's symptoms are hindered by:
Change of weather
Cold

Person's symptoms are helped by:
Rest
Lying down

Calc Phos

Bone health, builds cells, supports growth, restorative tonic

Body Part / System	Symptoms
Mind	exhaustion anxious about future impaired memory
Head	headaches especially during puberty dizziness / vertigo fontanelles remain open too long nosebleeds sinusitis pale complexion
Eyes	photophobia
Ears	ear ache and swollen glands
Mouth	tooth decay difficult teething inflamed gums sore aching throat chronic enlargement of tonsils
Digestive system	flatulence acidity, indigestion, heartburn gallstones
Respiratory system	bronchial asthma flu catarrh & tough stringy mucus suffocative cough
Kidneys/bladder	stones in bladder
Skin, blood & hair	acne hair loss following fever skin issues with thick yellow discharges general blood nutrient anaemia - helps provide new blood cells
Bones, joints & ligaments	general bone health broken bones & fractures arthritis, rheumatism with numb feeling sciatica
Female	amenorrhea (absent periods) uterine displacements

Calc Sulph
Number 1 blood cleanser

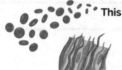

This salt is concentrated in:
Connective tissue
Blood
Liver bile

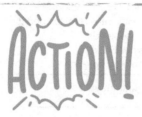

Blood purifier
Removes waste
Cleanses
Heals

GENERAL ACTION & KEYNOTES:

- Cleanses and purifies the body
- Helps with any ailment where the discharge process lasts too long
- Helps remove waste from the blood stream
- Speeds up wounds that are slow to heal (works well with Silica)
- Helps with any pus-forming ailment, e.g. boils
- Thick lumpy, yellow, pus-like discharges which may be blood streaked
- Glandular swellings, boils, abscesses, ulcers

ailments with pus

blood cleanser

boils, abscesses, swellings & ulcers

heals wounds

 warm water

 dry atmosphere

Person's symptoms are hindered by:
Washing in warm water
After waking
Being overheated

Person's symptoms are helped by:
Dry atmosphere

14

Calc Sulph

Blood cleanser, dissolves discharges, eliminates infections

Body Part / System	Symptoms
Mind	changeable mood irritable discontent sudden loss of memory
Head	acne edge of nostrils sore colds with thick discharges dandruff
Eyes	conjunctivitis (pink eye)
Ears	ear infections with bloody discharges
Mouth	tonsillitis where pus forms mouth ulcers
Digestive system	chronic constipation or diarrhoea
Respiratory system	bronchitis catarrh with thick, lumpy pus like secretions
Kidneys/bladder	kidney pain
Skin, blood & hair	any skin issue with pus - boils, ulcers & abscesses scaly skin acne liver spots glandular swellings chilblains cleanses blood & heals wounds
Bones, joints & ligaments	burning itching of soles of feet
Female	n/a

Ferrum Phos
Number 1 anti-inflammatory

This salt is concentrated in:
Haemoglobin of blood
Blood vessels
(Found in all body cells)

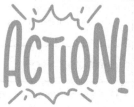

Anti-inflammatory
Transports oxygen
First Aid

GENERAL ACTION & KEYNOTES:

- Any inflammatory state and fevers
- Red, hot, swollen
- Use when 'feel like coming down with something'
- First stage of infection
- A disturbance of this salt can lead to congestion in the blood vessels causing increased blood pressure and risk of haemorrhage
- Helps with blood disorders and iron deficiency
- Oxygen carrier (in conjunction with Kali Sulph)
- Restores tone and equalises circulation
- Useful for low immunity

red & hot

'feel like coming down with something'

haemorrhage

blood disorders

 motion
 cold

Person's symptoms are hindered by:
Motion
Excitement
Warmth

Person's symptoms are helped by:
Cold
Slow motion

16

Ferrum Phos

First stage of illness, anti-inflammatory, oxygen transporter

Body Part / System		Symptoms
Mind		indifference tiredness & exhaustion
Head		rush of blood to head throbbing or catarrhal headache nosebleeds sinusitis
Eyes		eyes burning or sore sensation of grains of sand under eyelid
Ears		ear infection with burning or throbbing pain
Mouth		teething pain sore throat which is red and inflamed
Digestive system		diarrhoea with watery stools piles (hemorrhoids)
Respiratory system		first stage for colds bronchitis, pneumonia or flu acute asthma short, dry coughs or croup whooping cough with vomiting loss of voice or huskiness after singing lack of oxygen
Kidneys/bladder		frequent urination cystitis bedwetting
Skin, blood & hair		abscesses chicken pox, measles, mumps varicose veins anaemia haemorrhages high blood pressure
Bones, joints & ligaments		arthritis rheumatism sciatica sprains
Female		heavy periods

Kali Mur
Number 1 for congestion

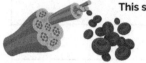 **This salt is concentrated in:**
Blood
Nerves
Muscles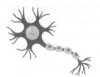

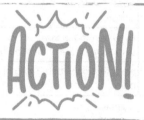

Detoxifies
Glandular tonic
Anti-congestion
Cleanses lymph

GENERAL ACTION & KEYNOTES:

- All second stage and chronic inflammations
- For any sluggish condition
- Useful for chronic catarrhal conditions, croup, diphtheria, pneumonia
- Helps eliminate thick, white, fatty discharges
- May have white/grey coating of tongue.
- Helps with any glandular issue
- Eliminates fatty build up in arteries
- Helps with production of saliva and thus can improve digestion

second stage inflammation

chronic catarrh

thick, white, discharges

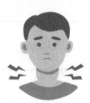
cleanses lymph

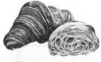
fatty food

Person's symptoms are hindered by:
Fatty food
Motion

Person's symptoms are helped by:
n/a

Kali Mur

Congestion, detoxifier, glandular tonic, lymph cleanser

Body Part / System	Symptoms
Mind	eating disorders
Head	congestion in glands & lymph nosebleeds sinusitis
Eyes	discharges of mucus ulcers of cornea
Ears	chronic catarrhal conditions of middle ear closed eustachian tubes ear infections, snapping noises in ear
Mouth	grey-white tongue coating thrush tonsillitis chronic sore throat coldsores & canker sores
Digestive system	diarrhoea with mucusy stools constipation vomiting & nausea sluggish liver
Respiratory system	catarrh and hawking of mucus loud, noisy cough with thick white discharge croup pneumonia or bronchitis asthma with white mucus
Kidneys/bladder	inflammation of bladder cystitis
Skin, blood & hair	abscesses where swelling but no pus acne chicken pox, measles, mumps eczema or skin issues with white discharges warts cleanses lymph
Bones, joints & ligaments	arthritis, rheumatism with swollen joints sciatica
Female	congestion in pelvic area

Kali Phos
Number 1 nerve tonic

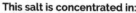

This salt is concentrated in:
Brain
Nerves
Muscles
Blood

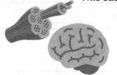
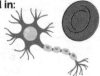

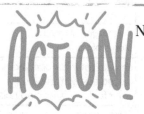

Nerve & brain nutrient
Calms nerves
Soothes
'Pick me up' tonic

GENERAL ACTION & KEYNOTES:

- Works directly on nerve tissues
- Aids healthy brain chemistry
- Helps with any condition arising from lack of nerve power, e.g. exhaustion, and burn out
- 'Pick me up' tonic
- Calms the entire system
- Useful for deep anxiety, nervous tension and emotional stress
- Lack of nerve tone such as twitches and weakness
- Helps aid a restful nights sleep

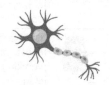

works on nerve tissues

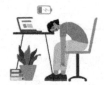

burnout

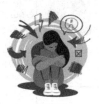

anxiety

insomnia

noise

gentle motion

Person's symptoms are hindered by:
Noise
Exertion
Cold air

Person's symptoms are helped by:
Gentle motion

Kali Phos

Nervousness, anxiety, fatigue

Body Part / System		Symptoms
Mind		exhaustion & burnout nervousness & anxiety brain fatigue from overwork depression /irritability weak memory & dementia insomnia
Head		nervous headaches worn out headache and due to overstudy sensitive to noise
Eyes		weak or distorted vision
Ears		buzzing sounds or twitching
Mouth		bleeding gums brown coating on tongue
Digestive system		hungry, all gone sensation diarrhoea caused by emotional upset 'butterflies' in tummy
Respiratory system		faintness and palpitations asthma with a depressed nervous state nervous asthma
Kidneys/bladder		n/a
Skin, blood & hair		itching of palms/soles high blood pressure
Bones, joints & ligaments		sciatica twitches & spasms
Female		amenorrhea (absent periods) pre-menstrual tension

Kali Sulph
Number 1 for skin issues

This salt is concentrated in:
Skin
Mucus membranes
Cell membranes

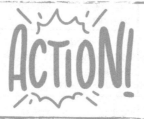

Conditions skin &
mucus membranes
Oxygen carrier

**GENERAL ACTION &
KEYNOTES:**

- Late/third stage inflammations
- Helps build new cells
- Helps eliminate any yellow-green discharges
- May have history of suppressing eruptions, e.g. steroid use
- For dry, scaly skin conditions
- Chronic catarrhal complaints
- Chronic discharges
- Lacks perspiration
- Works in conjunction with Ferrum Phos as an oxygen carrier
- Similar to the homeopathic remedy 'Pulsatilla'

**late stage
inflammations**

**yellow-green
discharges**

dry skin

chronic catarrh

 warm room **open air**

**Person's symptoms
are hindered by:**
Evening
Warm room

**Person's symptoms
are helped by:**
Open air

22

Kali Sulph

Skin issues, late stage infections, oxygen carrier

Body Part / System		Symptoms
Mind		irritable
Head		headache which is worse in warm room old catarrh causing lost sense of smell sinusitis
Eyes		failing vision
Ears		ear infections with yellow-green discharges deafness due to chronic catarrh
Mouth		burning thirst yellow slimy coating on tongue lost taste
Digestive system		may help with sugar cravings
Respiratory system		catarrh & mucous colds with yellow slimy matter asthma worse in warm season cough worse in evening or with yellow secretion rattling chest/cough whooping cough bronchitis suffocating feeling in warm rooms lack of oxygen
Kidneys/bladder		cystitis
Skin, blood & hair		any skin issues crusty/yellow greenish discharge eczema flaking/peeling skin liver spots athlete's foot ringworm brittle nails poor hair condition & dandruff
Bones, joints & ligaments		arthritis
Female		n/a

Mag Phos
Number 1 for cramps

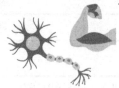

This salt is concentrated in:
Muscles
Nerves
Bone
Teeth
Blood

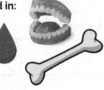

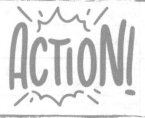

Anti-spasmodic
Nerve & muscle
relaxant

GENERAL ACTION & KEYNOTES:

- The #1 remedy for cramping as a lack of this salt causes contraction in muscle fibres
- Antispasmodic remedy so useful for issues such as stammering, twitches, tics, squinting, angina pains, hiccups, writer's cramps, dancer's cramp
- Colic
- Period pains that are helped by heat or pressure
- Helps with shooting or radiating pains
- Tension pains or headaches

cramping

shooting pain

period pains

tension headaches

 cold

 warmth

Person's symptoms are hindered by:
Cold

Person's symptoms are helped by:
Warmth
Pressure

Mag Phos

Cramps, pains, anti-spasmodic

Body Part / System		Symptoms
Mind		irritable insomnia
Head		spasmodic, pounding or tension headache relieved by application of warmth
Eyes		disturbed vision oversensitivity to light
Ears		ringing in ears deafness with anxiety
Mouth		teething
Digestive system		colic heartburn, indigestion hiccups diarrhoea with cramps piles (hemorrhoids) flatulence constipation gallstones
Respiratory system		whooping cough any spasmodic cough acute asthma
Kidneys/bladder		kidney stones spasmodic retention of urine
Skin, blood & hair		flushes
Bones, joints & ligaments		any cramps or muscle stiffness arthritis rheumatism sciatica
Female		period pains

Nat Mur
Balances fluid

 This salt is found in:
Every cell
and bodily fluid

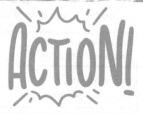 Water distributor
Fluid balancer
Regulates moisture
in the cells

**GENERAL ACTION &
KEYNOTES:**

- Attracts water to be used
  in the body (opposite of
  Nat Sulph which attracts
  water to eliminate)
- For any condition with
  excess or deficient fluid
- Distributes and balances
  fluid in the body
- Regulates moisture
- Helps any issue with clear
  watery discharges
- Dry skin
- Cracked lips
- Dehydration and dryness
- Salt deficiency
- Loss of taste and smell
- Craves salt

balances fluid

dryness

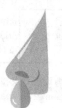
watery discharges

**loss of taste and
smell**

 :(**morning**

 :) **fresh air**

**Person's symptoms
are hindered by:**
Morning
Seaside

**Person's symptoms
are helped by:**
Fresh air

26

Nat Mur

Balances fluid, watery discharges, dryness, dehydration

Body Part / System		Symptoms
Mind		depressed - consolation aggravates tension & fatigue
Head		hammering headache especially with watery discharges sinusitis
Eyes		watery discharges granulated lids
Ears		roaring in ears watery discharges
Mouth		teething with lots of drooling cracks in corners of mouth sore throat with a feeling of a plug or lump dehydration coldsores & canker sores
Digestive system		constipation (dried out bowels) diarrhoea which alternates with constipation watery vomit waterbrash violent thirst yet longing for salt indigestion
Respiratory system		colds, catarrh & mucus - thin, watery discharges loss of taste and smell bronchitis asthma
Kidneys/bladder		bladder or kidney issues relieved by lying on back
Skin, blood & hair		eczema with clear discharges dry or cracking skin acne, warts anaemia hives
Bones, joints & ligaments		arthritis
Female		amenorrhea (absent periods)

Nat Phos
Acid neutraliser

This salt is concentrated in:
Brain
Blood
Bone
Muscles
Nerves

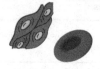

Neutralises acid
Balances acid

GENERAL ACTION & KEYNOTES:

- Regulates the balance of fats and acids in the body at all times
- A deficiency of this salt allows for uric acid to form leading to rheumatic symptoms
- Breaks down lactic acid
- Any issue due to excess acid, e.g. excess dairy, too many sweets, internal parasites
- Aids digestion
- Helps assimilate fats
- Helps insomnia due to to indigestion
- Golden yellow discharges or coating on tongue
- Sour discharges

natural 'ant-acid'

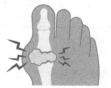

uric acid symptoms, e.g. gout

aids digestion

golden yellow tongue

😞 **morning**   🙂 **cold**

Person's symptoms are hindered by:
Morning
Fats

Person's symptoms are helped by:
Cold

28

Nat Phos

Acid neutraliser, balances acid

Body Part / System		Symptoms
Mind		anxious apprehensive fear insomnia
Head		headaches with gastric issues
Eyes		eyelids glued together in morning conjunctivitis (pink eye)
Ears		n/a
Mouth		thrush golden, yellow tongue
Digestive system		heartburn. indigestion, acidity grinding teeth pain after food diarrhoea with sour green stools vomiting sour fluids colic worms and parasites
Respiratory system		n/a
Kidneys/bladder		kidney stones cystitis
Skin, blood & hair		skin issues with yellow discharges greasy skin cradle cap hives
Bones, joints & ligaments		arthritis rheumatism gout all joint and muscle issues
Female		thrush any acidic vaginal secretions

Nat Sulph
Number 1 detoxifier

This salt is found concentrated in:
intercellular fluid

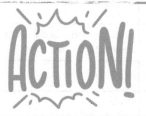

Diuretic
Regulates fluid
Skin conditioner
Stimulates liver

GENERAL ACTION:

- Attracts water to eliminate (opposite of Natrum Mur which attracts water to be used)
- Fluid retention especially in feet and legs
- Flushes toxic build up and eliminates excess water
- Helps heal gut
- Any liver related issues
- Useful for constipation especially when the individual feels 'cheerful after stool'
- Brown/green tongue
- Helps tone pancreas
- Use after head injury

eliminates water

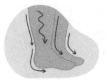

fluid retention

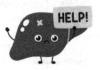

liver issues

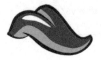

brown/green tongue

damp

warm, dry weather

Person's symptoms are hindered by:
Damp
Wet

Person's symptoms are helped by:
Warm, dry weather

Nat Sulph

Eliminates fluid, cleanses liver

Body Part / System	Symptoms
Mind	mental problems arising from head injury
Head	bilious headache head injuries
Eyes	n/a
Ears	n/a
Mouth	tongue looks dirty and green
Digestive system	bilious colic vomiting bile & nausea diarrhoea constipation - feels 'cheerful after stool' gallstones liver issues worse for lying on left side indigestion / heartburn persistent cough parasites and worms
Respiratory system	asthma worse in damp weather catarrh and green mucus cough with thick yellow-green mucus flu
Kidneys/bladder	supports kidney function diabetes sandy deposit in urine
Skin, blood & hair	eczema fluid retention cellulite
Bones, joints & ligaments	arthritis gout joint stiffness rheumatic pains worse for cold and damp
Female	genital itching

Silica
Skin and tissue conditioner

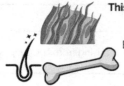

This salt is concentrated in:
Connective tissues
Hair & nails
Blood & blood vessels
Bile
Bone
Nerve cells

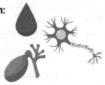

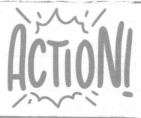

Cleanses and
conditions cells
Aids assimilation
Eliminates toxins

GENERAL ACTION:

- This salt is concentrated in connective tissues and acts prominently on bones, glands and skin
- Strengthens connective tissue
- Like a nutritional supplement aiding assimilation and metabolism
- Eliminates toxins
- Strengthens hair, skin and nails
- Slow healing or those who have tendency to scar
- Helps ripen and release abscesses (works well with Calc Sulph)

**strengthens
connective tissue**

**strengthens skin,
hair and nails**

aids elimination

ripens abscesses

Night

Heat

**Person's symptoms
are hindered by:**
Night
Full moon
Cold

**Person's symptoms
are helped by:**
Heat
Summer

Silica

Cell cleanser, skin and hair conditioner

Body Part / System		Symptoms
Mind		stronger mentally than physically oversensitive to noise
Head		chronic headaches sinusitis hair loss
Eyes		styes cataracts
Ears		can use when ear infection has turned to glue ear
Mouth		tooth decay canker sores sore gums or mouth
Digestive system		constipation especially where stools recede after having been partly expelled anal fissures poor assimilation of nutrients chronic diarrhoea
Respiratory system		slow healing infections such as pneumonia & bronchitis
Kidneys/bladder		chronic cystitis
Skin, blood & hair		abscesses & boils - helps ripen nails - cracked, ribbed, brittle & ingrown hair - loss, split ends, poor growth acne & pimples slow healing skin scars offensive sweating helps eliminate splinters
Bones, joints & ligaments		all skeletal strength problems arthritis rheumatism stiffness
Female		abscesses

Index of Symptoms

Index of Symptoms

Abscesses & boils
Calc Sulph
Ferrum Phos
Kali Mur
Silica

Acne
Calc Phos
Calc Sulph
Kali Mur
Nat Mur
Silica

Allergies
Kali Mur

Amenorrhea (absent periods)
Calc Phos
Kali Phos
Nat Mur

Anaemia
Calc Phos
Ferrum Phos
Nat Mur

Anxiety
Calc Phos
Kali Phos
Nat Phos

Arthritis
Calc Fluor
Calc Phos
Ferrum Phos
Kali Mur
Kali Sulph
Mag Phos
Nat Mur
Nat Phos
Nat Sulph
Silica

Asthma
Calc Phos
Ferrum Phos
Kali Mur
Kali Phos
Kali Sulph
Mag Phos
Nat Mur
Nat Sulph

Bladder issues
Calc Phos
Ferrum Phos
Kali Mur
Kali Sulph
Mag Phos
Nat Mur
Nat Phos
Nat Sulph

Broken bones
Calc Phos
Silica

Bronchitis
Calc Sulph
Ferrum Phos
Kali Mur
Kali Sulph
Nat Mur
Silica

Canker sores
Kali Mur
Nat Mur
Silica

Catarrh & mucus
Calc Phos
Calc Sulph
Ferrum Phos
Kali Mur
Kali Sulph
Nat Mur
Nat Sulph

Index of Symptoms

Cellulite
Nat Mur
Nat Sulph

Chicken pox
Ferrum Phos
Kali Mur

Colds
Calc Phos
Calc Sulph
Ferrum Phos
Kali Mur
Kali Sulph
Nat Mur

Coldsores
Calc Fluor
Kali Mur
Nat Mur

Colic
Mag Phos
Nat Phos
Nat Sulph

Constipation
Calc Fluor
Calc Sulph
Kali Mur
Mag Phos
Nat Mur
Nat Sulph
Silica

Coughs
Ferrum Phos
Kali Mur
Kali Sulph
Mag Phos
Nat Sulph

Cradle cap
Kali Sulph
Nat Phos

Cramps
Mag Phos

Croup
Calc Fluor
Ferrum Phos
Kali Mur
Mag Phos

Dandruff
Calc Sulph
Kali Sulph
Nat Mur

Diarrhoea
Calc Sulph
Ferrum Phos
Kali Mur
Kali Phos
Mag Phos
Nat Phos
Nat Sulph
Silica

Discharges
Calc Sulph (lumpy yellow)
Kali Mur (thick white)
Kali Sulph (yellow green)
Nat Mur (watery)
Nat Phos (golden yellow)

Ear issues
Calc Phos
Calc Sulph
Ferrum Phos
Kali Mur
Kali Sulph
Mag Phos
Silica

Eczema
Kali Mur
Kali Sulph
Nat Mur
Nat Sulph

36

Index of Symptoms

Exhaustion
Calc Phos
Ferrum Phos
Kali Phos

Eye issues
Calc Fluor
Calc Sulph
Ferrum Phos
Kali Mur
Kali Phos
Nat Mur
Nat Phos
Silica

Fevers
Ferrum Phos

Flatulence
Calc Phos
Mag Phos

Flu
Calc Phos
Ferrum Phos
Kali Mur
Kali Sulph
Nat Sulph

Gallstones
Calc Phos
Mag Phos
Nat Sulph

Glue ear
Silica

Gout
Nat Phos
Nat Sulph

Growing pains
Calc Phos
Mag Phos

Gum issues
Calc Fluor
Calc Phos
Silica

Hair loss
Calc Fluor
Calc Phos
Kali Sulph
Silica

Hayfever
Mag Phos
Nat Mur
Silica

Headaches
Calc Phos
Ferrum Phos
Kali Phos
Mag Phos
Nat Mur
Nat Phos
Nat Sulph
Silica

Hemorrhoids
Calc Fluor
Ferrum Phos
Mag Phos

Heartburn & indigestion
Calc Phos
Mag Phos
Nat Phos
Nat Sulph

Hiccups
Mag Phos

Hives
Kali Sulph
Nat Mur
Nat Phos

Index of Symptoms

Insomnia
Kali Phos
Mag Phos
Nat Phos

Joint issues
Calc Fluor
Calc Phos
Mag Phos
Nat Phos
Silica

Liver issues
Kali Mur
Nat Sulph

Measles
Ferrum Phos
Kali Mur
Kali Sulph

Mumps
Ferrum Phos
Kali Mur

Nausea
Kali Mur
Nat Phos

Nosebleeds
Ferrum Phos
Kali Mur

Palpitations
Calc Phos
Ferrum Phos
Mag Phos
Kali Phos
Nat Mur

Period pains
Calc Fluor
Calc Phos
Mag Phos

Pneumonia
Ferrum Phos
Kali Mur
Kali Phos
Silica

Prolapses
Calc Fluor

Rheumatism
Calc Phos
Ferrum Phos
Kali Mur
Mag Phos
Nat Phos
Nat Sulph
Silica

Sciatica
Calc Phos
Ferrum Phos
Kali Mur
Kali Phos
Mag Phos

Sinusitis
Calc Fluor
Calc Phos
Ferrum Phos
Kali Mur
Kali Sulph
Nat Mur
Silica

Skin issues
Calc Fluor
Calc Sulph
Kali Mur
Kali Sulph
Nat Mur
Nat Phos
Nat Sulph
Silica

Index of Symptoms

Sprains & strains
Calc Fluor
Calc Phos
Calc Sulph
Ferrum Phos
Mag Phos

Stretch marks
Calc Fluor

Sunstroke
Ferrum Phos
Nat Mur

Teething / toothache
Calc Fluor
Calc Phos
Ferrum Phos
Mag Phos
Nat Mur

Throat issues
Calc Fluor
Calc Phos
Calc Sulph
Ferrum Phos
Kali Mur
Nat Mur

Thrush (candida)
Kali Mur
Nat Mur
Nat Phos

Tooth decay
Calc Fluor
Calc Phos
Silica

Varicose veins
Calc Fluor
Ferrum Phos

Vertigo
Calc Phos
Ferrum Phos
Kali Phos
Nat Sulph

Vomiting
Kali Mur
Nat Mur
Nat Phos
Nat Sulph

Warts
Kali Mur
Nat Mur

Worms & parasites
Nat Sulph

Wounds
Calc Sulph
Ferrum Phos
Nat Sulph
Silica

Tissue Salt Combinations

Tissue salt combinations
'Make your own'

These tissue salts all work well together and have a synergetic effect. Make your own blend by administering the individual salts together

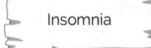

Insomnia

Nat Phos & Kali Phos Mag phos

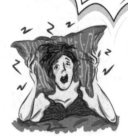

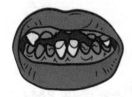

Tooth decay

Calc Phos & Calc Fluor Silica

Water retention

Nat Mur & Nat Sulph

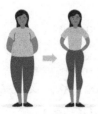

Weight loss

Calc Fluor & Calc Phos

Tissue salt combinations
'Standard combinations'

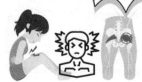

These are available pre-combined (denoted by the letters A, B, C etc) If you cannot find you can make your own by administering the individual salts together.

 a Neuralgia, sciatica, cramps & inflammation

Ferrum Phos, Kali Phos Mag Phos

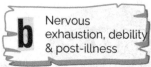 **b** Nervous exhaustion, debility & post-illness

Calc Phos, Kali Phos Ferrum Phos

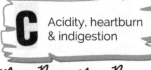 **c** Acidity, heartburn & indigestion

Mag Phos, Nat Phos, Nat Sulph, Silica

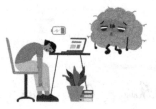

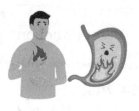

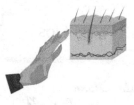 **d** Skin issues, eczema, dry skin & acne

Kali Mur, Kali Sulph Calc Sulph, Silica

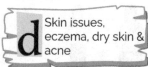

Tissue salt combinations
'Standard combinations'

These are available pre-combined (denoted by the letters A, B, C etc) If you cannot find you can make your own by administering the individual salts together.

 Tummy discomfort, bloating, gas, colic

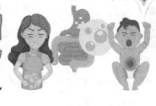

Calc Phos, Mag Phos, Nat Phos, Nat Sulph

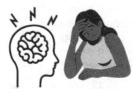

f Nervous headaches, migraines, weakness, fatigue

Kali Phos, Mag Phos, Nat Mur, Silica

 g Loss of elasticity, piles, backache

Calc Fluor, Calc Phos, Kali Phos, Nat Mur

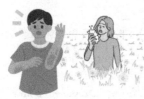

H Hayfever, allergies, rhinitis

Mag Phos, Nat Mur, Silica

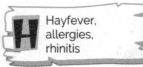

Tissue salt combinations
'Standard combinations'

These are available pre-combined (denoted by the letters A, B, C etc) If you cannot find you can make your own by administering the individual salts together.

 Muscular pains, inflammation

Ferrum Phos, Kali Sulph
Mag Phos

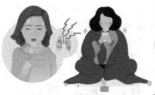

J Colds, chestiness, catarrh, coughs, flu. Use in winter

Ferrum Phos, Kali Mur
Nat Mur

 K Hair loss, brittle nails, flaky scalp

Kali Sulph, Nat Mur
Silica

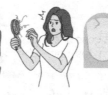

L Varicose veins, cold limbs, for those with a sedentary lifestyle

Calc Fluor, Ferrum Phos
Nat Mur

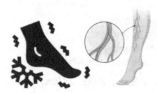 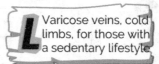

Tissue salt combinations
'Standard combinations'

These are available pre-combined (denoted by the letters A, B, C etc) If you cannot find you can make your own by administering the individual salts together.

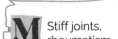 **M** Stiff joints, rheumatism

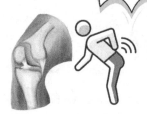

Calc Phos, Kali Mur
Nat Phos, Nat Sulph

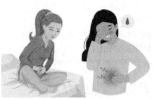

n Period pains, cramps

Calc Phos, Kali Mur
Kali Phos, Mag Phos

p Poor circulation, chillblains, aching feet & legs

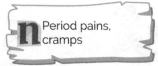

Calc Fluor, Calc Phos
Kali Phos, Mag Phos

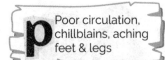

q Sinusitis, catarrh

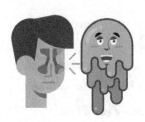

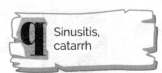

Ferrum Phos, Kali Mur
Kali Sulph, Nat Mur

45

Tissue salt combinations
'Standard combinations'

These are available pre-combined (denoted by the letters A, B, C etc) If you cannot find you can make your own by administering the individual salts together.

R Teething, tooth ache, dental inflammation

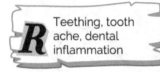

Calc Fluor, Calc Phos
Ferrum Phos, Mag Phos, Silica

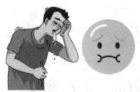

S Nausea, stomach upsets, biliousness

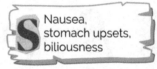

Kali Mur, Nat Phos
Nat Sulph

t First stage of minor illness

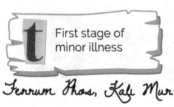

Ferrum Phos, Kali Mur

Ca Calcium

u Helps maximise calcium absorption

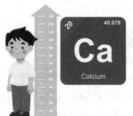

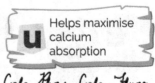

Calc Phos, Calc Fluor
Silica, Nat Phos

Tissue salt combinations
'Standard combinations'

These are available pre-combined (denoted by the letters A, B, C etc) If you cannot find you can make your own by administering the individual salts together.

(5) Contains the 5 phosphates.
Nerve tonic - For nerve issues, neuralgic pain, debility

Kali Phos, Mag Phos, Nat Phos
Calc Phos, Ferrum Phos

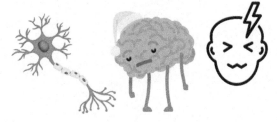

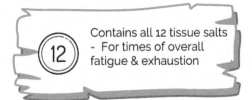

(12) Contains all 12 tissue salts - For times of overall fatigue & exhaustion

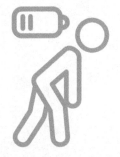

The Pregnancy Programme

The Pregnancy Programme
Summary

2nd month

Calc Fluor
for development of bones and
elasticity of connective tissue
helps prevent stretch marks, varicose
veins & piles

Mag Phos
for cramps and development of nerves

Ferrum Phos
for oxygenation of blood
stimulates absorption of iron

This is
a tried and tested 'protocol'
developed by the late
John Damonte, and is widely
used by homeopaths &
naturopaths to help support
their clients with a healthy
pregnancy.

3rd month

Calc Fluor
for development of bones and
elasticity of connective tissue
helps prevent stretch marks, varicose
veins & piles

Mag Phos
for cramps and development of nerves

Nat Mur
helps control fluid balance. and prevent
swollen ankles

Take one
tablet of each
tissue salt
morning and
evening of
each day.

4th month

Calc Fluor
for development of bones and
elasticity of connective tissue
helps prevent stretch marks, varicose
veins & piles

Nat Mur
helps control fluid balance. and prevent
swollen ankles

Silica
for teeth, bones, hair and general
strength, may also help with stretch
marks

The Pregnancy Programme
Summary

5th month

Calc Fluor
for development of bones and elasticity of connective tissue helps prevent stretch marks, varicose veins & piles

Ferrum Phos
for oxygenation of blood stimulates absorption of iron

Silica
for teeth, bones, hair and general strength, may also help with stretch marks

Take one tablet of each tissue salt morning and evening of each day.

6th month

Calc Fluor
for development of bones and elasticity of connective tissue helps prevent stretch marks, varicose veins & piles

Mag Phos
for cramps and development of nerves

Ferrum Phos
for oxygenation of blood stimulates absorption of iron

7th month

Calc Fluor
for development of bones and elasticity of connective tissue helps prevent stretch marks, varicose veins & piles

Mag Phos
for cramps and development of nerves

Nat Mur
helps control fluid balance. and prevent swollen ankles

51

The Pregnancy Programme
Summary

8th month

Calc Fluor

for development of bones and
elasticity of connective tissue
helps prevent stretch marks, varicose
veins & piles

Nat Mur

helps control fluid balance, and prevent
swollen ankles

Silica

for teeth, bones, hair and general
strength, may also help with stretch
marks

Take one
tablet of each
tissue salt
morning and
evening of
each day.

9th month

Calc Fluor

for development of bones and
elasticity of connective tissue
helps prevent stretch marks, varicose
veins & piles

Ferrum Phos

for oxygenation of blood
stimulates absorption of iron

Silica

for teeth, bones, hair and general
strength, may also help with stretch
marks

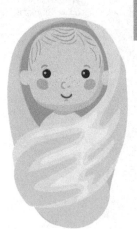

Relation of the Tissue Salts to the Zodiac Signs

Tissue Salts and the Zodiac Signs

George W. Carey was an American physician and author who wrote extensively about the relationship between tissue salts and astrology, particularly in his book 'The Relation of the Mineral Salts of the Body to the Signs of the Zodiac' (1932).

According to Carey's theory, each tissue salt corresponds to a specific astrological sign and deficiencies or imbalances in these salts may be influenced by astrological factors. For example, Carey suggested that individuals born under certain zodiac signs might be more prone to deficiencies in particular tissue salts, based on the astrological characteristics associated with their birth sign.

Carey's work delved into the symbolic and energetic qualities of both the tissue salts and the zodiac signs, drawing parallels between their respective properties. He proposed that by understanding the astrological correspondences of the tissue salts, one could gain insights into potential health issues or imbalances and take proactive measures to address them.

The table on the next page shows each zodiac sign, which body part/area is most likely to be afflicted and which tissue salt is likely to be of greatest benefit.

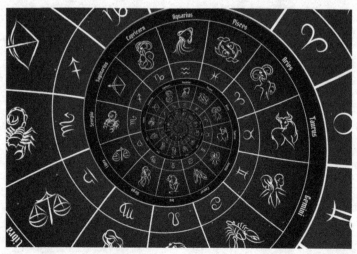

Tissue Salts and the Zodiac Signs

Zodiac sign	Tissue salt most likely to need	Areas most afflicted
Aries	Kali Phos	Brain - spinal cord - sensory nerves - lower jaw
Taurus	Nat Sulph	Liver - gallbladder - neck - throat - cerebellum
Gemini	Kali Mur	Lungs - glands - bronchi - shoulders - hands
Cancer	Calc Fluor	Breast - stomach - spleen - elastic tissue
Leo	Mag Phos	Heart - motor nerves - back
Virgo	Kali Sulph	Bowels - solar plexus
Libra	Nat Phos	Bladder - kidneys - acidity
Scorpio	Calc Sulph	Reproductive organs - vascular linings
Sagittarius	Silica	Hips - thighs - insulator
Capricorn	Calc Phos	Digestion - bones - knees - sacrum - blood proteins
Aquarius	Nat Mur	Ankles - blood plasma - white blood cells
Pisces	Ferrum Phos	Blood - red blood cells - feet

Your notes

My notes

My notes

My notes

My notes

My notes

Further reading

- Schuessler's Biochemic Pocket Guide with Repertory by W.H. Schuessler

- Schuessler's Twelve Tissue Remedies compliled and edited by William Boericke & W.A. Dewey

- The Relation of the Mineral Salts of the Body to the Signs of the Zodiac by George W. Carey

'Acid and alkali acting,
Proceeding and acting again.
Operating, transmuting, fomenting
In throes and spasms of pain -
Uniting, reacting, creating,
Like souls 'passing under the rod'-
Some people call it Chemistry,
And others call it God '

George W. Carey

About Lisa Strbac

LCHE BSc(Hons)

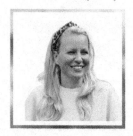

I'm a certified Homeopath LCHE BSc (Hons) and an ambassador for my profession. I'm passionate about empowering the individual to take responsibility for their own health, with the understanding that true health comes from within. Learning how to use homeopathy and tissue salts in the home is one of the most transformational steps an individual can make for their own and their family's health.

My journey towards holistic health started in 2015, after witnessing the power of homeopathy to heal my then 5 year old daughter's chronic autoimmune condition. I was a previous sceptic but I had exhausted all conventional approaches. I was so awestruck with homeopathy that I had to learn more, and, after 4 years of study and clinical practice, I obtained my Licentiate from the UK's largest accredited college, The Centre for Homeopathic Education. I am also an Integrative Nutrition Health Coach, having studied at The Institute of Integrative Nutrition, the world's largest health coaching and nutrition school.

My 'work' has evolved to teaching individuals on how to use homeopathy at home and I run a variety of very popular homeopathy online courses, which my attendees have described as 'life changing.' If every individual had a basic homeopathy kit and knew how to use it, the world would be a very different place.

We could avoid so many health issues if we understood how to naturally support health rather than suppress symptoms - homeopathy is amazing for this and there really is nothing else out there quite like it.

For more information on me and my courses you can connect with me at **www.lisastrbac.com.**

Lisa Strbac

By the same author:

The Homeopath in Your Hand - 77 remedies and how to select them using Homeopathy HEALS ™

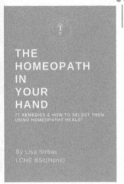

THE HOMEOPATH IN YOUR HAND

77 REMEDIES & HOW TO SELECT THEM USING HOMEOPATHY HEALS

By Lisa Strbac
LCHE BSc(Hons)

"
Learning how to use homeopathy in the home is one of the most empowering and transformational steps an individual can make towards improving their health.

The author, Lisa Strbac, has run popular homeopathy courses to thousands of people and has been asked consistently by attendees to create a book based on her 'life changing' courses. This book covers what are the most essential remedies to have at home including 'combination' remedies to have on hand in case you get stuck or are unsure what to give.

Each remedy is summarised in a clear and concise manner with beautiful illustrations helping to bring each one to life. In total, this book guides you through 77 single/combination remedies along with the foundations of homeopathy including how to select a remedy using the Homeopathy HEALS method taught by Lisa in her courses.
"

Reviews

⭐⭐⭐⭐⭐

A total gamechanger! The Homeopathy book we've been waiting for
Finally a homeopathy book for the home user that has everything in one place. Until now I've had to use multiple books but now I don't need to. Each remedy is illustrated and covers key symptoms, modalities, mental symptoms and aetiologies. I love the way the author has explained how to select a remedy using her Homeopathy HEALS technique. This book is a gamechanger!

My new favourite This is the clearest homeopathic home prescriber book I own/have browsed through. I love that I no longer need to cross reference 3-4 books and a pile of screenshots to choose a remedy. It's straight to the point and very friendly to the eye, the many little illustrations help to grasp and memorise the key points of the remedy even quicker.

Easy, accessible, idiot proof handbook on how to treat self and family naturally - AWESOME book! Clear instructional information. Little bit of background to homeopathy and how it works. Lists 77 remedies that are considered to be the most important ones. A great tool for empowering yourself in how to heal issues

Beautiful book - I don't normally leave reviews but this book deserves one !! It's beautifully presented , easy to read and understand. A great book if you're new to homeopathy or already knowledgeable. I cannot recommend highly enough.

This book is AMAZING. So easy to follow, full beginners instructions, cheaper than booking a homeopathy appointment…Lisa you have smashed it. This book is going to fly into the world and change lives.

Now this is going to change home prescribing forever.

⭐⭐⭐⭐⭐

Made in the USA
Monee, IL
06 October 2024

67303695R00046